PROLOG

Female Pelvic Medicine and Reconstructive Surgery

Assessment Book

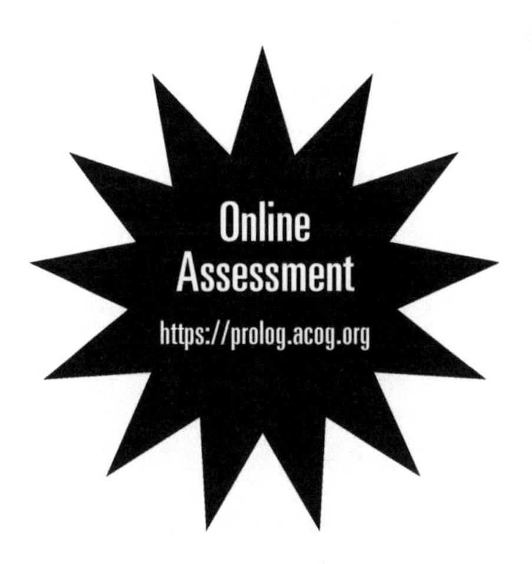

The American College of Obstetricians and Gynecologists
WOMEN'S HEALTH CARE PHYSICIANS

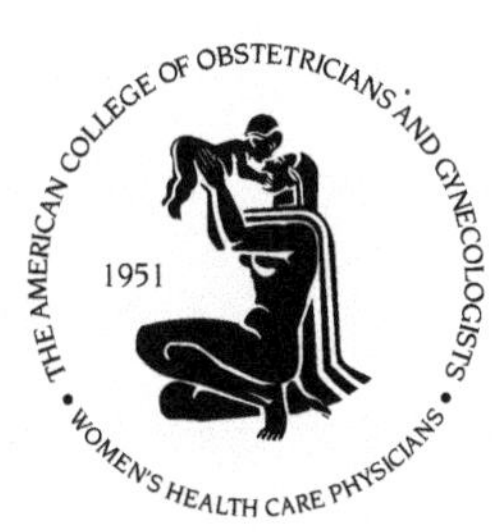

ISBN 978-1-948258-23-4

45/0

The American College of Obstetricians and Gynecologists
409 12th Street, SW
PO Box 96920
Washington, DC 20090-6920

Contributors

PROLOG Editorial and Advisory Committee

CHAIR

Ronald T. Burkman Jr, MD
Professor of Obstetrics and Gynecology
Department of Obstetrics and Gynecology
Tufts University School of Medicine
Baystate Medical Center
Springfield, Massachusetts

MEMBERS

Louis Weinstein, MD
Past Paul A. and Eloise B. Bowers Professor and Chair
Department of Obstetrics and Gynecology
Thomas Jefferson University
Philadelphia, Pennsylvania

PROLOG Task Force for *Female Pelvic Medicine and Reconstructive Surgery*

CHAIR

Kimberly Kenton MD, MS
Chief and Fellowship Program Director
Division of Female Pelvic Medicine & Reconstructive Surgery
Departments of Obstetrics & Gynecology and Urology
Northwestern University Feinberg School of Medicine
Chicago, Illinois

MEMBERS

Melinda G. Abernethy, MD, MPH
Assistant Professor
Division of Female Pelvic Medicine and Gynecologic Surgery
Department of Gynecology and Obstetrics
Johns Hopkins Hospital
Baltimore, Maryland

Jennifer Anger, MD, MPH
Associate Professor of Urology
Associate Director of Urological Research
Urologic Reconstruction, Urodynamics, and Female Urology
Cedars-Sinai Medical Center
Beverly Hills, California

Cara Grimes, MD, MAS
Assistant Professor of Obstetrics and Gynecology
Female Pelvic Medicine and Reconstructive Surgery
Gynecologic Specialty Surgery
Columbia University Medical Center
New York, New York

Catherine Matthews, MD
Professor
Department of Obstetrics & Gynecology and Urology
Wake Forest Baptist Health
Winston Salem, North Carolina

Continued on next page

PROLOG Task Force for *Female Pelvic Medicine and Reconstructive Surgery (continued)*

Olga Ramm, MD
Division of Female Pelvic Medicine and Reconstructive Surgery
Department of Obstetrics and Gynecology
Kaiser Permanente East Bay
The Permanente Medical Group
Oakland, California

COLLEGE STAFF

Sandra A. Carson, MD
Vice President for Education
Erica Bukevicz, MBA, MS
Senior Director, Educational Development and Testing
Division of Education
Christopher T. George, MLA
Editor, PROLOG
Anne Arnold, MA
Education Programs Director

CONFLICT OF INTEREST DISCLOSURE

This PROLOG unit was developed under the direction of the PROLOG Advisory Committee and the Task Force for *Female Pelvic Medicine and Reconstructive Surgery*. PROLOG is planned and produced in accordance with the Standards for Enduring Materials of the Accreditation Council for Continuing Medical Education. Any discussion of unapproved use of products is clearly cited in the appropriate critique.

Current guidelines state that continuing medical education (CME) providers must ensure that CME activities are free from the control of any commercial interest. The task force and advisory committee members declare that neither they nor any business associate nor any member of their immediate families has material interest, financial interest, or other relationships with any company manufacturing commercial products relative to the topics included in this publication or with any provider of commercial services discussed in the unit. All potential conflicts have been resolved through the American College of Obstetricians and Gynecologists' mechanism for resolving potential and real conflicts of interest.

Preface

Purpose

PROLOG (Personal Review of Learning in Obstetrics and Gynecology) is a voluntary, strictly confidential self-evaluation program. PROLOG was developed specifically as a personal study resource for the practicing obstetrician–gynecologist. It is presented as a self-assessment mechanism that, with its accompanying performance information, should assist the physician in designing a personal, self-directed lifelong learning program. It may be used as a valuable study tool, a reference guide, and a means of attaining up-to-date information in the specialty. The content is carefully selected and presented in multiple-choice questions that are clinically oriented. The questions are designed to stimulate and challenge physicians in areas of medical care that they confront in their practices or when they work as consultant obstetrician–gynecologists.

PROLOG also provides the American College of Obstetricians and Gynecologists (the College) with one mechanism to identify the educational needs of the Fellows. Individual scores are reported only to the participant; however, cumulative performance data and evaluation comments obtained for each PROLOG unit help determine the direction for future educational programs offered by the College.

Process

The PROLOG series offers the most current information available in five areas of the specialty: obstetrics, gynecology and surgery, reproductive endocrinology and infertility, gynecologic oncology and critical care, and patient management in the office. A new PROLOG unit is produced annually, addressing one of those subject areas. The College also produces volumes of PROLOG that concentrate on additional specialty areas, such as *Female Pelvic Medicine and Reconstructive Surgery.*

Each unit of PROLOG represents the efforts of a task force of subject experts under the supervision of an advisory committee. PROLOG sets forth current information as viewed by recognized authorities in the field of women's health. This educational resource does not define a standard of care, nor is it intended to dictate an exclusive course of management. It presents recognized methods and techniques of clinical practice for consideration by obstetrician–gynecologists to incorporate in their practices. Variations of practice that take into account the needs of the individual patient, resources, and the limitations that are special to the institution or type of practice may be appropriate.

Each unit of PROLOG is presented as a two-part set, with performance information and cognate credit available to those who choose to submit their answers electronically for confidential scoring. Participants can work through the unit at their own pace, choosing to use PROLOG as a closed or open assessment. The Critique Book provides the rationale for correct and incorrect options, and current, accessible references.

Continuing Medical Education Credit

ACCME Accreditation

The American College of Obstetricians and Gynecologists is accredited by the Accreditation Council for Continuing Medical Education (ACCME) to provide continuing medical education for physicians.

AMA PRA Category 1 Credit(s)™

The American College of Obstetricians and Gynecologists designates this enduring material for a maximum of 14 ***AMA PRA Category 1 Credits***™. Physicians should claim only the credit commensurate with the extent of their participation in the activity.

College Cognate Credit(s)

The American College of Obstetricians and Gynecologists designates this enduring material for a maximum of 14 Category 1 College Cognate Credits. The College has a reciprocity agreement with the American Medical Association that allows *AMA PRA Category 1 Credits™* to be equivalent to College Cognate Credits.

Participants who submit their assessment and achieve a passing score will be credited with 14 hours and will receive a Performance Report that provides a comparison of their scores with the scores of a sample group of physicians who have taken the unit as an examination. An individual may request credit only once for each unit.

Credit for PROLOG *Female Pelvic Medicine and Reconstructive Surgery* is initially available through December 2018. During that year, the unit will be reevaluated. If the content remains current, credit is extended for an additional 3 years, with credit for the unit automatically withdrawn after December 2021.

New: Electronic Assessment for CME Credit

For this unit, the CME Assessment can only be submitted electronically. Assessment results must be above 80% to achieve a passing score and attain CME credit. To access the online assessment, please visit www.acog.org/PROLOGexam. Test results and the CME certificate will be available upon completion of the examination.

If you purchased a print book, use the key code located on the inside front cover of the Critique Book and follow the directions provided. If you purchased an eBook, please follow the instructions online to purchase and access the assessment.

Conclusion

PROLOG was developed specifically as a personal study resource for the practicing obstetrician–gynecologist. It is presented as a self-assessment mechanism that, with its accompanying performance information, should assist the physician in designing a personal, self-directed learning program. The many quality resources developed by the College, as detailed each year in the College's *Publications and Educational Materials Catalog*, are available to help fulfill the educational interests and needs that have been identified. PROLOG is not intended as a substitute for the certification or recertification programs of the American Board of Obstetrics and Gynecology.

PROLOG CME SCHEDULE

Gynecologic Oncology and Critical Care, Sixth Edition	Credit through 2016
Patient Management in the Office, Sixth Edition	Reevaluated in 2014–Credit through 2017
Obstetrics, Seventh Edition	Reevaluated in 2015–Credit through 2018
Gynecology and Surgery, Seventh Edition	Reevaluated in 2016–Credit through 2019
Reproductive Endocrinology and Infertility, Seventh Edition	Reevaluated in 2017–Credit through 2020
Gynecologic Oncology and Critical Care, Seventh Edition	Reevaluated in 2018–Credit through 2021
Female Pelvic Medicine and Reconstructive Surgery	Reevaluated in 2018–Credit through 2021

PROLOG Objectives

PROLOG is a voluntary, strictly confidential, personal continuing education resource that is designed to be stimulating and enjoyable. By participating in PROLOG, obstetrician–gynecologists will be able to do the following:

- Review and update clinical knowledge.
- Recognize areas of knowledge and practice in which they excel, be stimulated to explore other areas of the specialty, and identify areas requiring further study.
- Plan continuing education activities in light of identified strengths and deficiencies.
- Compare and relate present knowledge and skills with those of other participants.
- Obtain continuing medical education credit, if desired.
- Have complete personal control of the setting and of the pace of the experience.

The obstetrician–gynecologist who completes *Female Pelvic Medicine and Reconstructive Surgery* will be able to

- discuss normal pelvic anatomy and physiology and how alterations in anatomy and physiology contribute to development of pelvic floor disorders.
- identify the pathophysiologic and epidemiologic factors that contribute to pelvic floor disorders in women.
- associate symptom bother and quality of life effect of different pelvic floor disorders, determine appropriate diagnostic workups, and select accurate diagnoses.
- associate pelvic floor symptoms with corresponding signs on examination and testing to ensure accurate diagnoses.
- discuss the alternative surgical and nonsurgical treatment options for pelvic floor disorders and identify common complications of therapy.
- apply knowledge of anatomy and appropriate surgical techniques in the surgical treatment of pelvic floor disorders.

Female Pelvic Medicine and Reconstructive Surgery includes the following topics:

SCREENING AND DIAGNOSIS
Nerve entrapment with uterosacral ligament suspension
Office evaluation of incontinence
Pelvic anatomy
Rectal prolapse
Spinal cord lesion
Stress urinary incontinence
Vaginal agenesis
Vertebral discitis

MEDICAL MANAGEMENT
Aging and hormonal effects on the pelvic floor
Bowel complications after robotic sacrocolpopexy
Cystoscopy
Detrusor sphincter dyssynergia
Fecal incontinence
Mesh complications
Midurethral slings
Neuromodulation for urgency urinary incontinence
Nocturia
Occult stress incontinence in patient with prolapse

Painful bladder syndrome
Pelvic mesh materials
Pelvic organ prolapse
Posthysterectomy fistula
Rectovaginal fistula
Recurrent urinary tract infection
Sacrospinous ligament suspension complications
Stress urinary incontinence
Upper limb nerve injury
Urgency urinary incontinence
Urinary diversion
Urinary incontinence treatment options
Urinary retention
Venous thromboembolism and perioperative thromboprophylaxis
Wound breakdown

PHYSIOLOGY
Ectopic ureter
Lower limb peripheral nerve injury
Pelvic anatomy
Pelvic organ prolapse quantification
Rectal prolapse
Urethral diverticula

SURGICAL MANAGEMENT
Apical prolapse
Electrosurgery
Intraoperative cystoscopy
Lower limb peripheral nerve injury
Pelvic organ prolapse repair
Posterior vaginal wall prolapse
Risk factors for obstetric laceration
Upper limb nerve injury
Urethral diverticula
Use of the POP-Q test to determine surgical options

EPIDEMIOLOGY AND BIOSTATISTICS
Lower limb peripheral nerve injury

COUNSELING
Botulinum toxin for urgency urinary incontinence
Mesh complications
Mode of delivery and pelvic floor dysfunction
Stress urinary incontinence

ETHICAL AND LEGAL ISSUES
Surgical proctoring

OFFICE PROCEDURES
Office evaluation of incontinence

A complete subject matter index appears at the end of the Critique Book.

Instructions for Taking the Electronic Assessment

For this unit, the CME Assessment can only be submitted electronically. Assessment results must be above 80% to achieve a passing score and attain CME credit. To access the online assessment, please visit www.acog.org/PROLOGexam. Test results and the CME certificate will be available upon completion of the examination.

Use the key code located on the inside front cover of the Critique Book and follow the directions provided. If you do not wish to submit your answers for scoring, you will not receive credit. The Critique Book enclosed in this package will, however, enable you to score your own examination.

DIRECTIONS: Each of the questions or incomplete statements below is followed by suggested answers or completions. Select the ONE that is BEST in each case, and fill in the circle containing the corresponding letter on the answer sheet.

1

A 17-year-old girl comes to your office for evaluation of a vaginal wall cyst that had been noted by her primary care provider. She is asymptomatic and has no comorbidities. She is not sexually active and reports regular menses. She experienced menarche at age 12 years. Pelvic examination reveals a painless, fluctuant, fluid-filled 6-cm mass on the left lateral vagina, approximately 4 cm cephalad to the hymenal ring (Fig. 1-1). The most likely diagnosis is

(A) urethral diverticulum
(B) mesonephric duct remnant
(C) Bartholin cyst
(D) pronephric duct remnant
(E) Skene gland cyst

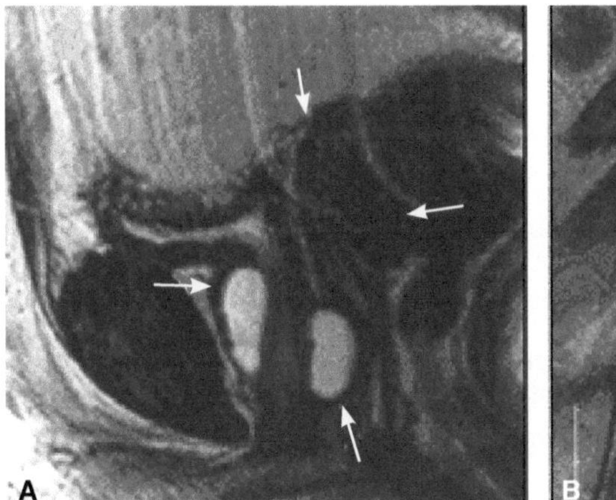

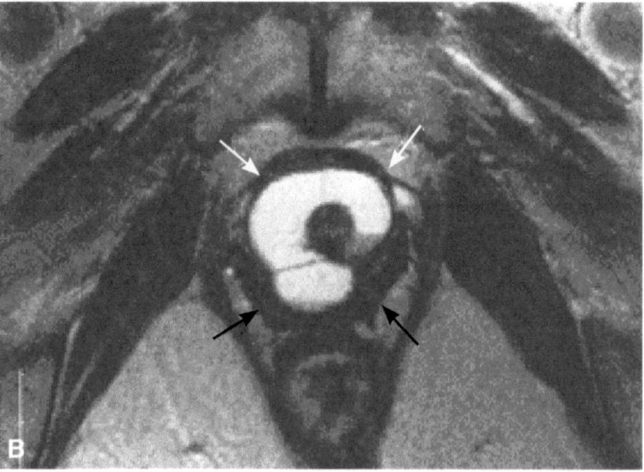

FIG. 1-1. Urethral diverticulum as seen on magnetic resonance imaging. (Reprinted with permission of Anderson Publishing Ltd. from Hubert J, Bergin D. Imaging the female pelvis: when should MRI be considered? Appl Radiol 2008;37:9–24. Copyright Anderson Publishing, Ltd.)

2

A 65-year-old woman, gravida 3, para 3, has stage III anterior vaginal wall prolapse. The surgical repair that is most likely to resolve her underlying pelvic support defect is

(A) anterior repair with midline plication
(B) anterior repair with insertion of polypropylene mesh
(C) bilateral paravaginal repair
(D) anterior repair with sacrospinous ligament fixation

Note: See Appendix A for a table of normal values for laboratory tests.

3

A 30-year-old woman, gravida 1, para 0, at 28 weeks of gestation, asks for your advice in regard to mode of delivery. She is contemplating a cesarean delivery by maternal request because she is concerned about pelvic floor dysfunction. You advise her that the immediate postpartum risk that cesarean delivery may help to reduce is

(A) urinary incontinence
(B) anal incontinence
(C) pelvic organ prolapse
(D) levator spasms

4

A primiparous woman comes to your office 10 days postpartum after a forceps-assisted vaginal delivery with a third-degree tear. She reports increased perineal pain and bleeding. On examination, she is found to have complete breakdown of her wound with no evidence of infection (Fig. 4-1; see color plate). The most appropriate management strategy is to

(A) allow healing by secondary intention
(B) prescribe oral antibiotics and re-examine in 1 week
(C) perform prompt surgical repair in the operating room
(D) perform closure in the office

5

A 35-year-old obese Hispanic woman had a second stage of labor that was 3 hours in duration. Her infant was in the persistent occiput posterior position. She underwent a forceps-assisted vaginal delivery with midline episiotomy. On delivery, the infant weighed 3,856 g (8.5 lb). The greatest risk of anal sphincter injury during this delivery was

(A) midline episiotomy
(B) forceps-assisted delivery
(C) infant weight
(D) persistent occiput posterior position
(E) Hispanic ethnicity

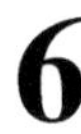

A 71-year-old woman is referred to you for symptoms of urinary tract infection, which have improved after a 3-day course of antibiotics. Her dipstick urinalysis is positive for leukocyte esterase and negative for blood. Urine culture is positive for *Escherichia coli*. She has had three culture-proven urinary tract infections over the past 2 years. She recalls that she had one to two urinary tract infections while in her twenties. She is sexually active with one long-term partner. On pelvic examination, she has no structural abnormalities and has stage I pelvic organ support. The best next step in management is

(A) computed tomography (CT) urography
(B) antibiotic suppression
(C) cystoscopy
(D) vaginal estrogen
(E) renal ultrasonography

7

A 71-year-old multiparous woman visits your office with a symptomatic vaginal bulge. She noticed the bulge after her total vaginal hysterectomy 2 years ago, and it has become progressively more bothersome. On examination, she has stage III pelvic organ prolapse. She has a total vaginal length of 10 cm, and her vaginal cuff protrudes past the hymen; however, it is not completely everted (Fig. 7-1; see color plate). The correct pelvic organ prolapse quantification (POP-Q) assessment for this patient is

(A)

–2	–2	–8
3	2	10
–1	–1	–10

(B)

–3	–3	–8
3	2	10
–3	–3	X

(C)

+3	+6	+6
3	2	10
–1	+6	X

(D)

+3	+6	+6
3	2	10
–1	+6	+4

(E)

+3	+10	+10
3	2	10
+3	+10	X

8

A 54-year-old woman comes to your office with urinary incontinence that has worsened over the past year. She reports leaking with coughing, sneezing, or laughing (two to three times per day), which requires a minipad. She also notes rare incontinence associated with a feeling of urgency. She does not have any bulge symptoms or bowel concerns. A standing cough stress test is carried out, during which small drops of urine are seen leaking from her urethra when she coughs. Her pelvic organ prolapse quantification test results are as follows:

–2	–2	–6
4	3	10
–2	–2	–5

Her urethra is hypermobile with excursion from 10 degrees to 85 degrees with straining. After sending a urine sample for culture and sensitivity, the best next step in her evaluation is

(A) wait for culture results
(B) obtain a postvoid residual urine volume
(C) multichannel urodynamic testing
(D) dynamic magnetic resonance imaging
(E) midurethral sling surgery

9

A 46-year-old woman, para 2, reports urinary incontinence that is intermittent throughout the day and night and has become more severe over the past 4 months. She describes leaking when running to the bathroom, after sneezing, and when getting out of the car after a long trip. She notes waking up once or twice at night with a strong desire to void and leaking on the way to the toilet. You elicit a medical history and perform multichannel cystometrography (Fig. 9-1; see color plate). The best next step in management is

(A) incontinence ring pessary
(B) periurethral bulking injection
(C) fluid intake modulation and timed voiding
(D) pelvic floor physical therapy
(E) trial of sacral neuromodulation

10

A 62-year-old obese woman has a diagnosis of mixed urinary incontinence after her workup. She does not want to undergo a surgical procedure but desires to try behavioral interventions. Along with pelvic floor muscle exercises, the intervention that is most likely to reduce leakage is

(A) weighted vaginal cones
(B) incontinence pessary
(C) elimination of caffeine
(D) modest weight loss

11

A 32-year-old woman, gravida 1, para 1, comes to your clinic with urinary incontinence. She hopes to become pregnant within the next year. She reports that after delivery of her son 8 months ago, she developed urine leakage with exercise, and specifically with running. The leakage interferes with her quality of life. She has no symptoms of urgency urinary incontinence. The best treatment option for her is

(A) incontinence dish pessary
(B) urethral bulking
(C) bladder neck fascial sling
(D) synthetic midurethral sling
(E) anticholinergic medication

12

A 44-year-old woman, gravida 3, para 3, comes to your office and reports that she leaks urine with coughing, sneezing, and jogging. On examination, she has a positive cough stress test. She is interested in undergoing surgical treatment and recently heard about retropubic midurethral slings. You counsel her that the most common complication associated with a retropubic midurethral sling procedure is

(A) bladder perforation
(B) hemorrhage
(C) neurologic symptoms
(D) persistent voiding dysfunction
(E) urinary tract infection

13

A 42-year-old woman visits your clinic with urinary incontinence. She first developed urinary leakage with exercise, coughing, and sneezing after delivery of her first child. She has completed her family and desires surgical management. She does not report symptoms of urgency or urgency incontinence. She voids seven times per day, and has no prolapse or vaginal bulge. Her postvoid residual urine volume is 55 mL, and urine culture is negative. The most important test in the evaluation of this patient for surgery is

(A) urodynamic testing
(B) cough stress test
(C) ultrasonography
(D) cystoscopy
(E) computed tomography urography

14

A 55-year-old woman comes to your office with urgency incontinence. She states that she experiences five or six daily episodes of large-volume urine loss associated with an urge to void. She also reports enuresis with involuntary urination at night. She uses six to seven incontinence pads per day. She has tried behavioral therapy, including timed voiding and decreasing bladder irritants. She most recently tried two anticholinergic medications with no improvement in symptoms. She decides to try an intradetrusor injection of onabotulinumtoxinA. You counsel her that this is a very effective therapy but is accompanied by a high rate of urinary tract infections and the adverse effect of

(A) dry eye
(B) nausea
(C) urinary retention
(D) leg weakness and numbness
(E) psychosis

15

A 65-year-old woman has daily episodes of urgency urinary incontinence, despite the fact that she has reduced her fluid intake and performs Kegel exercises correctly. She requires one to two incontinence pads daily. She tried oxybutynin chloride three times a day with good success initially. However, she developed adverse effects (dry mouth, dry eyes, and constipation), which led her to stop using the medication. Her primary care provider is currently performing a workup for episodic hypertension. The next best step is to prescribe

(A) mirabegron once daily
(B) oxybutynin chloride XL once daily
(C) oxybutynin XL twice daily
(D) tolterodine tartrate twice daily

16

An 84-year-old woman visits your office with urgency urinary incontinence. She reports five to six daily episodes of large-volume urine loss associated with an urge to void. She wears multiple incontinence pads per day and feels unable to leave her house for long periods because of the need for frequent pad and clothing changes. She has tried behavioral therapy, including timed voiding and decreasing bladder irritants. She has narrow-angle glaucoma and is unable to tolerate anticholinergic medications. Her postvoid residual urine volume in the office is 200 mL. She has elected to pursue a trial of sacral neuromodulation. She had a permanent lead placed adjacent to the S3 dorsal root and is working on a daily bladder diary. Her diary today shows a greater than 50% improvement in her urinary leakage episodes. The most appropriate next step is to

(A) pull the lead
(B) replace the external battery pack
(C) acupuncture
(D) place a permanent neurostimulator
(E) pursue percutaneous stimulation of the tibial nerve

17

A woman develops leakage per vagina on postoperative day 2 after a laparoscopic hysterectomy. Her surgery involved some intraoperative bleeding at the vaginal cuff, which was controlled with suture ligation, and she went home after she voided on postoperative day 1. She was prescribed oral phenazopyridine to confirm that the fluid was urine, and there was orange fluid on her pad. She underwent an office cystoscopy on postoperative day 3, which revealed a 0.5-cm × 0.5-cm defect in the bladder posterior to the trigone and 1 cm posterior to the trigone and medial to the right ureteral orifice. The best next step in management is

(A) indwelling Foley catheter for 2–3 weeks
(B) renal scan with furosemide
(C) computed tomography urography
(D) immediate operative repair of fistula
(E) renal ultrasonography

18

As part of the hospital credentialing requirements, each surgeon must perform two proctored surgical cases. Your chairman requests that you serve as a surgical proctor for a new physician in the process of obtaining privileges. A surgical proctor would not be expected to

(A) receive institutional compensation for proctoring
(B) teach a new faculty surgeon certain portions of the procedure
(C) complete written evaluation of the new faculty surgeon
(D) recommend termination of the procedure if the patient is at risk

19

A 77-year-old woman, para 4, is undergoing vaginal hysterectomy and bilateral salpingo-oophorectomy with uterosacral ligament suspension for the treatment of stage 3 pelvic organ prolapse. You suspend the anterior and posterior vaginal cuff to the uterosacral ligaments bilaterally using delayed absorbable suture. After administering intravenous (IV) dye, you perform cystoscopy and fail to see urine efflux from either the left or right ureteral orifice. The best next step in management is

(A) administer an IV fluid bolus
(B) administer IV furosemide
(C) insert open-ended stents
(D) remove the uterosacral suspension sutures

20

An 87-year-old multiparous woman with multiple medical comorbidities comes to your office for evaluation of pelvic organ prolapse noted during her recent hospitalization for myocardial infarction. She reports no typical prolapse symptoms but has urinary incontinence. On examination, her anterior vaginal wall is prolapsed 6 cm beyond the hymen, and her cervix is at the hymen. You obtain a postvoid residual urine volume, which is 260 mL. Urinalysis is negative for nitrites, leukocytes, and blood. The best next step in her management is

(A) indwelling Foley catheter
(B) antimuscarinic medication
(C) prolapse reduction with pessary
(D) urodynamic testing
(E) colpocleisis and rectus fascial sling

21

A healthy 35-year-old woman, para 2, comes to your office 6 weeks after uncomplicated placement of a retropubic midurethral sling. She reports urinary frequency, a slow dribbling urinary stream, and a sensation of incomplete bladder emptying. Her stress urinary incontinence symptoms have resolved after surgery. She reports no dysuria or hematuria. Her postvoid residual urine volume is 340 mL and her urine dipstick is negative. She is using self-catheterization. The most appropriate management of her condition is

(A) trial of bethanechol
(B) pelvic floor therapy
(C) surgical sling lysis
(D) recheck postvoid residual urine volume after 6 weeks of self-catheterization
(E) insertion of a suprapubic catheter

22

A 42-year-old woman reports urinary leaking with exercise, coughing, and sneezing after the delivery of her child 10 years ago. She has had no leakage associated with an urge to void. For the past few years, she has successfully used an incontinence dish, but she has decided that she is finished with childbearing and wants to pursue definitive surgical management. She underwent an uncomplicated transobturator midurethral polypropylene sling procedure. Cystoscopy at the time of the procedure revealed intact bladder and urethra with bilateral ureteral efflux. Six months after her sling surgery, she is happy that she can now exercise without leaking urine. However, she notes intermittent vaginal spotting between her menses and her partner describes "something scratchy" during intercourse. Figure 22-1 (see color plate) shows your findings on pelvic examination. You advise her that the most appropriate next step is

(A) observation
(B) prescribe estrogen cream
(C) surgically remove the entire sling
(D) place a cadaver fascia sling over the existing sling

23

A 65-year-old sexually active woman desires surgical management of her stage III pelvic organ prolapse. The vaginal bulge interferes with her daily activities, and she sometimes has difficulty emptying her bladder. She does not have symptoms of stress or urgency urinary incontinence. She experiences three episodes of nocturia each night. Her postvoid residual urine volume is 175 mL. She wants a procedure that will offer the best anatomic and functional outcome. The best next treatment for this patient is

(A) sacrocolpopexy with Burch colposuspension
(B) sacrocolpopexy without Burch colposuspension
(C) colpocleisis with rectus fascial sling
(D) colpocleisis without rectus fascial sling
(E) sacrospinous ligament suspension with midurethral sling

24

A 57-year-old woman comes to your office with a 6-month history of urinary urgency and frequency plus bladder pain. She has been treated for recurrent urinary tract infections but reports negative urine cultures. On examination, she has pain with insertion of the speculum and bladder tenderness on bimanual examination. Otherwise, her pelvic examination is normal. Her urinalysis is negative. The most appropriate next step in management is

(A) office cystoscopy
(B) potassium sensitivity test
(C) pelvic floor physical therapy
(D) pentosan polysulfate
(E) amitriptyline

25

A 70-year-old woman with a history of chronic obstructive pulmonary disease has had recurrent urinary tract infections every 2 months for the past year. All of her urinary tract infections have been culture proved, and her symptoms have resolved each time with the use of antibiotics. She is not sexually active and has been taking vaginal estrogen for 6 months. She was given a prescription for once-daily trimethoprim–sulfamethoxazole but developed a resistant urinary tract infection after 3 months of therapy. Office-based cystoscopy is negative. Her urine appears cloudy, and she has a postvoid residual urine volume of 100 mL. After ruling out an active urinary tract infection, the best next treatment is

(A) cranberry pills plus vitamin C
(B) methenamine hippurate plus vitamin C
(C) nitrofurantoin monohydrate
(D) increase vaginal estrogen to three times weekly

26

A 63-year-old woman comes to your office with a vaginal bulge that she felt over the past year. She has had to push on this bulge to complete urination and defecation. She has no significant previous medical history and has never undergone surgery. She experienced menopause at age 51 years and has had no postmenopausal bleeding. She is sexually active. On examination, she has an intact sacral nerve. Her levator ani muscles are weak, with only a flicker of a squeeze felt on your fingers during examination. Her anterior vaginal wall reduces with support of the cervix with a large procto swab. Her uterus is small and mobile. Her pelvic organ prolapse quantification (POP-Q) test is as follows:

+3	+5	+6
4	3	10
–1	–1	+4

The best surgical option to correct her prolapse is

(A) Burch colposuspension
(B) anterior and posterior colporrhaphy
(C) abdominal sacrocolpopexy
(D) vaginal hysterectomy
(E) placement of vaginal mesh

27

A 63-year-old woman with anterior predominant pelvic organ prolapse comes to your office for a second opinion regarding surgery for pelvic organ prolapse. A surgeon has recommended an anterior colporrhaphy with synthetic mesh augmentation. She is considering proceeding with this surgery but would like to discuss possible complications associated with vaginal mesh. You inform her that the most likely complication after vaginal placement of synthetic mesh is

(A) pelvic or vaginal pain
(B) dyspareunia
(C) recurrent prolapse
(D) vaginal infection
(E) mesh exposure

28

A 45-year-old woman comes to your office with symptomatic stage III pelvic organ prolapse. She has been using a pessary for the past 5 years, but now she desires surgical management. She is an avid triathlete, and she recently completed her first Ironman race. She does not report any urinary or bowel symptoms and is sexually active. Her apex and anterior vaginal wall are 5 cm outside the hymen. She desires the most durable repair with the quickest recovery time. The most appropriate surgical procedure for her is

(A) sacrospinous ligament suspension
(B) laparoscopic sacrocolpopexy
(C) uterosacral ligament suspension
(D) colpocleisis
(E) iliococcygeus suspension

29

Pelvic organ prolapse repair sometimes is augmented with an implantable reconstructive material to improve the durability of the reconstruction. The characteristic of the pelvic mesh that results in the lowest rate of mesh extrusion is

(A) microporous (less than 10 microns)
(B) high density
(C) low elasticity
(D) monofilament
(E) nonabsorbable

30

A patient who underwent robotic sacrocolpopexy 4 days ago has nausea, vomiting, and cramping abdominal pain. On examination, she appears ill and has a tender, distended abdomen. The most appropriate initial management strategy is

(A) exploratory laparotomy
(B) abdominal flat plate
(C) computed tomography (CT) scan with contrast
(D) diagnostic laparoscopy

31

A 73-year-old woman has had a vaginal bulge for 6 months. She has not experienced urinary incontinence or retention, and she reports no bowel concerns. She has diabetes mellitus and hypertension controlled with medications. She has had reconstructive pelvic surgery, including uterosacral ligament suspension. At the same time, she received a total vaginal hysterectomy and bilateral salpingo-oophorectomy. She has tried a pessary but is unable to retain one because of poor levator tone and a wide genital hiatus. On examination, her pelvic organ prolapse quantification test result is as follows:

–2	+3	+5
5	2	8
+1	+1	

She desires surgical correction and chooses to undergo a sacrospinous ligament suspension. During the procedure, after placement of two permanent sutures one fingerbreadth medial to the ischial spine along the sacrospinous ligament, brisk bleeding is encountered. The bleeding is controlled with application of topical thrombin and prolonged application of manual pressure. The sutures are then affixed to the vaginal mucosa in the standard fashion to complete the apical repair. A posterior colporrhaphy and perineorrhaphy then are performed with excellent reduction of the prolapse. In the recovery room, the patient immediately complains of severe right-sided buttock pain that radiates down the back of her leg. The best next step in management is

(A) observation
(B) evacuation of suspected hematoma
(C) release of sacrospinous sutures
(D) proctoscopy with removal of posterior repair and perineorrhaphy sutures

32

A 13-year-old adolescent girl is brought to your office by her mother with reports of urinary incontinence. She experiences continuous leakage of a small amount of urine during the day and overnight. She otherwise voids normally several times a day and does not have urinary urgency, frequency, or dysuria. Renal ultrasonography demonstrates a duplicated left collecting system and vaginoscopy shows a left ureteric opening into the vaginal vault. The embryonic structure that is the result of this abnormal development is the

(A) mesonephric duct
(B) metanephric blastema
(C) paramesonephric duct
(D) urogenital sinus
(E) pronephros

33

A 17-year-old girl comes to your office with primary amenorrhea. She reports breast development at age 12 years and no cyclic pelvic pain. On examination, she has Tanner stage 4 breasts. Her external genitalia appear normal with the exception of a vaginal dimple. Ultrasonography fails to visualize a uterus. The initial laboratory test to confirm her diagnosis is her level of

(A) follicle-stimulating hormone (FSH)
(B) luteinizing hormone (LH)
(C) prolactin
(D) testosterone
(E) dehydroepiandrosterone sulfate

34

A 35-year-old woman with a history of spinal cord injury undergoes a cystoscopy as part of her workup for recurrent urinary tract infections. On filling the bladder to approximately 400 mL, she suddenly develops a headache and sweating on her face. Her blood pressure is 180/100 mm Hg and her heart rate is 45 beats per minute. The bladder is emptied, the cystoscope is removed, and symptoms immediately resolve. The patient likely has a spinal cord lesion located at

(A) cord level T4
(B) cord level T8
(C) spinal column level T6
(D) spinal column level T8

35

A 48-year-old woman, para 1, with a symptomatic 5-cm urethral diverticulum requests surgical management. She also reports bothersome stress urinary incontinence. Office cystometry demonstrates urinary leakage with cough and Valsalva, 200 mL bladder volume, and maximum urethral closure pressure of 18 cm H_2O. The best concomitant anti-incontinence procedure for this patient is

(A) periurethral bulking injection
(B) retropubic midurethral sling
(C) transobturator midurethral sling
(D) laparoscopic Burch urethropexy
(E) autologous fascial sling

36

A 58-year-old stress-continent woman has a body mass index (weight in kilograms divided by height in meters squared [kg/m^2]) of 22 and stage III pelvic organ prolapse. She undergoes an uncomplicated open supracervical hysterectomy, sacrocolpopexy, and Burch colposuspension. The surgery is done in the dorsal lithotomy position through a Pfannenstiel incision using a Balfour retractor and lasts 3 hours. On postoperative day 1, she falls as she is trying to get out of bed. She had decreased motor strength of her left quadriceps muscle (2/5), sensory loss over the anterior thigh, and an absent patellar reflex. Based on her symptoms, the nerve that has most likely been injured is

(A) femoral
(B) obturator
(C) sciatic
(D) common peroneal
(E) ilioinguinal

37

A 65-year-old multiparous female comes to your office with accidental bowel leakage. She reports several loose stools per day with associated leakage. She has a history of anal sphincter laceration with her first delivery 40 years ago. The intervention that is most likely to eliminate her fecal incontinence is

(A) overlapping anal sphincteroplasty
(B) loperamide
(C) sacral neuromodulation
(D) biofeedback
(E) posterior levatorplasty

38

A 30-year-old healthy woman visits your office with gas and loose stool per vagina 4 weeks after fourth-degree repair after a vaginal delivery. She is found to have a 7-mm rectovaginal fistula above the anal sphincter complex. The most appropriate management is

(A) temporary diverting colostomy
(B) expectant management for 3 months
(C) mobilization of fistula tract and layered closure
(D) fibrin plug
(E) high-fiber diet

39

A 48-year-old woman with stage III uterovaginal prolapse is scheduled for a robotic-assisted laparoscopic supracervical hysterectomy and abdominal sacrocervicopexy followed by perineorrhaphy and placement of a midurethral sling. Before the procedure, she is positioned on the table with foam padding to secure her torso, along with shoulder rests to assure that she does not slip up the table while she is in a steep Trendelenburg position. The hysterectomy is difficult because of a uterine fibroid and multiple adhesions that require an additional 30 minutes of lysis of adhesions. The entire surgical procedure lasted 6 hours. During rounds the next day, the patient tells you that she is unable to pick up her coffee cup with her right hand, although she has no pain. The best next step in management is

(A) observation
(B) thoracic magnetic resonance imaging
(C) physical therapy
(D) neuropathic pain medication
(E) surgical reattachment of the affected nerve

40

An 82-year-old woman, para 4, with nighttime urinary urgency and frequency tells you that she is awakened four to five times every night with the need to go to the toilet. She experiences urinary incontinence on occasion, despite “running to the bathroom.” She does not have bothersome urinary symptoms during the daytime. In addition to keeping a voiding diary, you tell her that the best next step is

(A) oral desmopressin
(B) bedside commode for nighttime use
(C) intradetrusor botulinum toxin A injection
(D) oral oxybutynin at bedtime
(E) percutaneous tibial nerve stimulation

41

An 80-year-old woman who underwent colpocleisis 1 year ago comes to your office with intermittent fecal incontinence. She reports a sensation of incomplete bowel evacuation and rectal fullness. The most likely finding on physical examination is

(A) prolapsing internal hemorrhoids
(B) rectal prolapse
(C) posterior wall prolapse
(D) rectal intussusception

42

A 35-year-old woman had a diving accident 2 years ago, resulting in a complete T9 spinal cord injury. Immediately after the accident, she developed acute urinary retention requiring an indwelling urethral catheter. After she recovered from her injuries, she was taught clean intermittent catheterization, which she performed without any issues until 1 year after the accident, at which time she developed urinary incontinence between catheterizations. Her incontinence was controlled with anticholinergic agents for nearly 12 months. However, more recently, she has developed progressively worse leakage between catheterizations. Urodynamic tests demonstrate poor compliance, with detrusor pressure increasing to 50 cm H_2O at a volume of 150 mL and a detrusor leak point pressure of 60 cm H_2O at a volume of 200 mL. She has no leakage with cough or Valsalva maneuver. Renal ultrasonography reveals mild bilateral hydronephrosis. The best next step in management is

(A) increase anticholinergic agents
(B) increase rate of clean intermittent catheterization
(C) ileocystoplasty
(D) augmentation cystoplasty with continent cutaneous stoma
(E) ileal conduit urinary diversion

43

A 50-year-old woman was diagnosed with multiple sclerosis after an episode of acute urinary retention. She was initially managed with an indwelling catheter for 2 weeks, after which she was taught clean intermittent catheterization. Three months later, she regained the ability to void again and was fully continent. However, over the next 6 months she developed voiding difficulty with periodic leakage in which she totally emptied her bladder in her wheelchair. At her office visit, her postvoid residual urine volume was 400 mL. She returned to the office 1 week later for urodynamic testing. Before emptying her with a catheter, her initial postvoid residual urine volume was 450 mL. Her urodynamic testing demonstrates the tracing illustrated in Figure 43-1 (see color plate). The best next step in management for her is

(A) augmentation cystoplasty
(B) indwelling Foley catheter
(C) clean intermittent catheterization and anticholinergic agent
(D) suprapubic tube placement

44

A 52-year-old woman is undergoing a midurethral retropubic synthetic sling placement for stress urinary incontinence. Immediately after trocar placement, gross hematuria is noted in the Foley catheter. With the use of a 70-degree lens, cystoscopy is performed and reveals bilateral perforations of the sling trocars. The passers then are removed. Repeat cystoscopy reveals ongoing brisk bleeding from the left-sided trocar site, resulting in red-colored urine. The best next step is

(A) abandon the sling procedure
(B) replace the sling
(C) continuous bladder irrigation for 48 hours
(D) abdominal repair by cystotomy

45

A 58-year-old woman comes to your office with a vaginal bulge that she has felt for the past year. In order to defecate, she has to use her fingers to push on her perineum and inside her vagina. She tells you, "It feels like my stool is getting stuck." She has not experienced bowel leakage. She has no significant prior medical history and has never had surgery. She is sexually active. She had a forceps delivery of a 3,629-g (8-lb) infant and recalls a tear into her rectum. A rectovaginal examination demonstrates a distal pocket and laxity. She desires definitive surgical management. On examination, her pelvic organ prolapse quantification test result is as follows:

–2	–2	–7
4	2	10
+3	+4	–8

You recommend

(A) posterior colporrhaphy
(B) graft-augmented site-specific posterior vaginal wall repair
(C) sacral colpoperineopexy
(D) transanal rectocele repair

46

A 45-year-old woman comes to the emergency department 5 months after undergoing a robotic-assisted laparoscopic sacrocolpopexy. She reports back pain and lower extremity pain and weakness. On examination, she is afebrile with tenderness over the lumbosacral spine and normal neurologic function. Spinal magnetic resonance imaging reveals increased L5–S1 vertebral body and intervertebral disc enhancement on T2 weighted images. The most likely microbial pathogen associated with her vertebral discitis is

(A) *Candida albicans*
(B) group B *Streptococcus*
(C) *Mycobacterium tuberculosis*
(D) *Pseudomonas aeruginosa*
(E) *Staphylococcus aureus*

47

A 74-year-old woman visits your office with a vaginal bulge she has felt for 6 months. She has experienced no urinary incontinence, retention, or bowel issues. She has no prior surgical history and has well-controlled diabetes mellitus. On examination, she has stage III uterine prolapse. She tried a pessary but did not like the maintenance required and instead has elected to undergo definitive surgical correction. After options counseling, she chooses to have a total vaginal hysterectomy with bilateral salpingo-oophorectomy and uterosacral ligament suspension. Postoperatively, she is experiencing pain and numbness in the left buttock that radiates down the back of her thigh to her popliteal fossa. No motor compromise is detected. The most likely cause of her pain and numbness is

(A) compression of the common peroneal nerve
(B) entrapment of sacral nerve roots
(C) femoral neuropathy
(D) diabetic neuropathy

48

During a laparoscopic salpingo-oophorectomy, you use a bipolar electrosurgical energy source to secure the blood supply to the ovary within the infundibulopelvic ligament before transecting it. The correct term for the electrosurgical function you perform with the bipolar device is

(A) cauterization
(B) fulguration
(C) vaporization
(D) coagulation

49

A 57-year-old postmenopausal woman comes to your clinic for preoperative counseling. She has stage III uterovaginal prolapse and is scheduled to undergo a vaginal hysterectomy and uterosacral ligament suspension. Her weight is 90.7 kg (200 lb), and her body mass index (weight in kilograms divided by height in meters squared [kg/m^2]) is 37. She is otherwise healthy, has no history of venous thromboembolism, does not smoke, and takes combination hormone therapy. Based on the patient's presentation, her perioperative thromboprophylaxis should be

(A) early ambulation
(B) compression stockings
(C) intermittent pneumatic compression devices
(D) enoxaparin twice daily

50

A 42-year-old multiparous woman has urinary leakage with coughing, sneezing, and exercise. She tried an incontinence pessary in the past without improvement in her symptoms. Her anterior vaginal wall comes to the hymen and she has urethral hypermobility. Her cough stress test result is positive. After discussing the nonsurgical and surgical options, she is eager for definitive management and wants the treatment with highest success rate and shortest recovery time. The most appropriate treatment for this patient is

(A) autologous fascial sling
(B) onabotulinumtoxinA
(C) midurethral sling
(D) urethral bulking agent
(E) physical therapy

PROLOG USER DEMOGRAPHICS AND PROLOG EVALUATION

To obtain a profile of the group of Fellows choosing to use self-assessment as a continuing medical education tool, the Education Division would appreciate the following information. This is for education program planning only and will not be associated with score reports in any way.

D1. Which describes your main area of practice?

(A) Obstetrics only
(B) Gynecology only
(C) Obstetrics and Gynecology
(D) Do not provide patient care (office only)

D2. Which best describes your main practice model?

(A) Solo practice
(B) Ob-gyn group
(C) Multispecialty group
(D) Medical school/univeristy/teaching hospital
(E) Military/government
(F) Staff model HMO
(G) Other:____________________

D3. Please select which of the following PROLOG formats you purchased:

(A) eBook PROLOG only
(B) Print copy PROLOG only
(C) Both the PROLOG eBook and PROLOG print copy
(D) Not applicable

D4. In the future, I will

(A) purchase both the PROLOG eBook and PROLOG print copy formats of an edition.
(B) purchase the PROLOG eBook only.
(C) purchase the PROLOG print copy only.
(D) not purchase any editions of PROLOG.

D5. Compared with mailing a paper assessment to ACOG, I prefer completing the assessment online.

(A) Strongly agree
(B) Somewhat agree
(C) Somewhat disagree
(D) Strongly disagree
(E) I have never completed a paper assessment.

D6. The functionality and overall design of the new online assessment were easy to use and fulfilled my expectations for completing the assessment.

(A) Strongly agree
(B) Somewhat agree
(C) Somewhat disagree
(D) Strongly disagree

D7. Other comments I have regarding this edition of PROLOG and the online assessment:

____

____

____

____

____

____

____

____

____

____

Appendix A

Normal Values for Laboratory Tests*

Analyte	Conventional Units
Alanine aminotransferase, serum	8–35 units/L
Alkaline phosphatase, serum	15–120 units/L
Menopause	
Amniotic fluid index	3–30 mL
Amylase	20–300 units/L
Greater than 60 years old	21–160 units/L
Aspartate aminotransferase, serum	15–30 units/L
Bicarbonate	
Arterial blood	21–27 mEq/L
Venous plasma	23–29 mEq/L
Bilirubin	
Total	0.3–1 mg/dL
Conjugated (direct)	0.1–0.4 mg/dL
Newborn, total	1–10 mg/dL
Blood gases (arterial) and pulmonary function	
Base deficit	Less than 3 mEq/L
Base excess, arterial blood, calculated	–2 mEq/L to +3 mEq/L
Forced expiratory volume (FEV_1)	3.5–5 L
	Greater than 80% of predicted value
Forced vital capacity	3.5–5 L
Oxygen saturation (Sao_2)	95% or higher
Pao_2	80 mm Hg or more
Pco_2	35–45 mm Hg
Po_2	80–95 mm Hg
Peak expiratory flow rate	Approximately 450 L/min
pH	7.35–7.45
Pvo_2	30–40 mm Hg
Blood urea nitrogen	
Adult	7–18 mg/dL
Greater than 60 years old	8–20 mg/dL
CA 125	Less than 34 units/mL
Calcium	
Ionized	4.6–5.3 mg/dL
Serum	8.6–10 mg/dL
Chloride	98–106 mEq/L
Cholesterol	
Total	
Desirable	140–199 mg/dL
Borderline high	200–239 mg/dL
High	240 mg/dL or more
High-density lipoprotein	40–85 mg/dL
Low-density lipoprotein	
Desirable	Less than 130 mg/dL
Borderline high	140–159 mg/dL
High	Greater than 160 mg/dL
Total cholesterol-to-high-density lipoprotein ratio	
Desirable	Less than 3
Borderline high	3–5
High	Greater than 5
Triglycerides	
20 years and older	Less than 150 mg/dL
Younger than 20 years old	35–135 mg/dL

*Values listed are specific for adults or women, if relevant, unless otherwise differentiated.

(continued)

Normal Values for Laboratory Tests* *(continued)*

Analyte	Conventional Units
Cortisol, plasma	
8 AM	5–23 micrograms/dL
4 PM	3–15 micrograms/dL
10 PM	Less than 50% of 8 AM value
Creatinine, serum	0.6–1.2 mg/dL
Dehydroepiandrosterone sulfate	60–340 micrograms/dL
Erythrocyte	
Count	3,800,000–5,100,000/mm^3
Distribution width	10 plus or minus 1.5%
Sedimentation rate	
Wintrobe method	0–15 mm/hour
Westergren method	0–20 mm/hour
Estradiol-17β	
Follicular phase	30–100 pg/mL
Ovulatory phase	200–400 pg/mL
Luteal phase	50–140 pg/mL
Child	0.8–56 pg/mL
Ferritin, serum	18–160 micrograms/L
Fibrinogen	150–400 mg/dL
Follicle-stimulating hormone	
Premenopause	2.8–17.2 mIU/mL
Midcycle peak	15–35 mIU/mL
Postmenopause	24–170 mIU/mL
Child	0.1–7 mIU/mL
Glucose	
Fasting	70–105 mg/dL
2-hour postprandial	Less than 120 mg/dL
Random blood	65–110 mg/dL
Hematocrit	36–48%
Hemoglobin	12–16 g/dL
Fetal	Less than 1% of total
Hemoglobin A_{1c} (nondiabetic)	5.5–8.5%
Human chorionic gonadotropin	0–5 mIU/mL
Pregnant	Greater than 5 mIU/mL
17α-Hydroxyprogesterone	
Adult	50–300 ng/dL
Child	32–63 ng/dL
25-Hydroxyvitamin D	10–55 ng/mL
International Normalized Ratio	Greater than 1
Prothrombin time	10–13 seconds
Iron, serum	65–165 micrograms/dL
Binding capacity total	240–450 micrograms/dL
Lactate dehydrogenase, serum	313–618 units/L
Leukocytes	
Total	5,000–10,000/cubic micrometers
Differential counts	
Basophils	0–1%
Eosinophils	1–3%
Lymphocytes	25–33%
Monocytes	3–7%
Myelocytes	0%
Band neutrophils	3–5%
Segmented neutrophils	54–62%

*Values listed are specific for adults or women, if relevant, unless otherwise differentiated.

(continued)

Normal Values for Laboratory Tests* (*continued*)

Analyte	Conventional Units
Lipase	
60 years or younger	10–140 units/L
Older than 60 years	18–180 units/L
Luteinizing hormone	
Follicular phase	3.6–29.4 mIU/mL
Midcycle peak	58–204 mIU/mL
Postmenopause	35–129 mIU/mL
Child	0.5–10.3 mIU/mL
Magnesium	
Adult	1.6–2.6 mg/dL
Child	1.7–2.1 mg/dL
Newborn	1.5–2.2 mg/dL
Mean corpuscular	
mCH Hemoglobin	27–33 pg
mCHC Hemoglobin concentration	33–37 g/dL
mCV Volume	80–100 cubic micrometers
Partial thromboplastin time, activated	21–35 seconds
Phosphate, inorganic phosphorus	2.5–4.5 mg/dL
Platelet count	140,000–400,000/mm^3
Potassium	3.5–5.3 mEq/L
Progesterone	
Follicular phase	Less than 3 ng/mL
Luteal phase	2.5–28 ng/mL
On oral contraceptives	0.1–0.3 ng/mL
Secretory phase	5–30 ng/mL
Older than 60 years	0–0.2 ng/mL
1st trimester	9–47 ng/mL
2nd trimester	16.8–146 ng/mL
3rd trimester	55–255 ng/mL
Prolactin	0–17 ng/mL
Pregnant	34–386 ng/mL by 3rd trimester
Prothrombin time	10–13 seconds
Reticulocyte count	Absolute: 25,000–85,000 cubic micrometers 0.5–2.5% of erythrocytes
Semen analysis, spermatozoa	
Antisperm antibody	% of sperm binding by immunobead technique; greater than 20% = decreased fertility
Count	Greater than or equal to 20 million/mL
Motility	Greater than or equal to 50%
Morphology	Greater than or equal to 15% normal forms
Sodium	135–145 mEq/L
Testosterone, female	
Total	6–86 ng/dL
Pregnant	3–4 × normal
Postmenopause	One half of normal
Free	
20–29 years old	0.9–3.2 pg/mL
30–39 years old	0.8–3 pg/mL
40–49 years old	0.6–2.5 pg/mL
50–59 years old	0.3–2.7 pg/mL
Older than 60 years	0.2–2.2 pg/mL
Thyroid-stimulating hormone	0.2–3 microunits/mL
Thyroxine	
Serum free	0.9–2.3 ng/dL
Total	1.5–4.5 micrograms/dL

*Values listed are specific for adults or women, if relevant, unless otherwise differentiated.

(continued)

Normal Values for Laboratory Tests* (*continued*)

Analyte	Conventional Units
Triiodothyronine uptake	25–35%
Urea nitrogen, blood	
Adult	7–18 mg/dL
Older than 60 years	8–20 mg/dL
Uric acid, serum	2.6–6 mg/dL
Urinalysis	
Epithelial cells	0–3/HPF
Erythrocytes	0–3/HPF
Leukocytes	0–4/HPF
Protein (albumin)	
Qualitative	None detected
Quantitative	10–100 mg/24 hours
Pregnancy	Less than 300 mg/24 hours
Urine specific gravity	
Normal hydration and volume	1.005–1.03
Concentrated	1.025–1.03
Diluted	1.001–1.01

*Values listed are specific for adults or women, if relevant, unless otherwise differentiated.

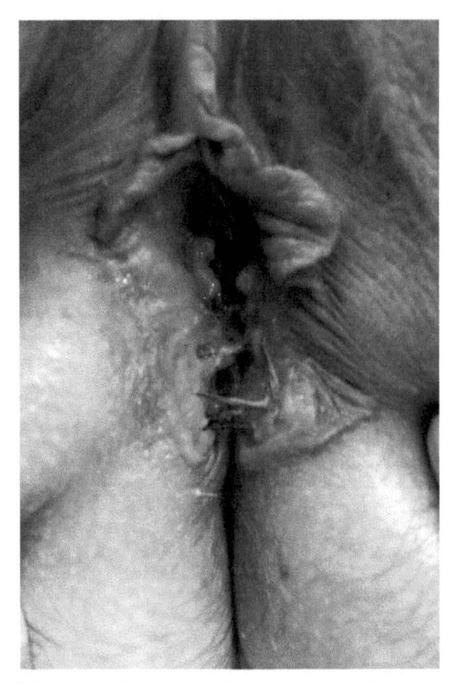

FIG. 4-1. Complete breakdown of wound. (Courtesy of Catherine Matthews, MD.)

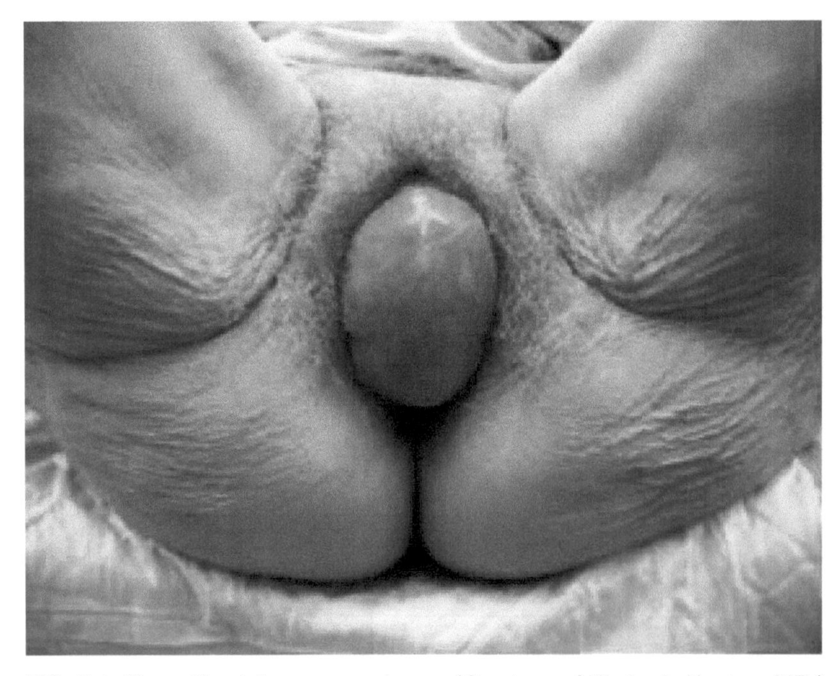

FIG. 7-1. Stage III pelvic organ prolapse. (Courtesy of Kimberly Kenton, MD.)

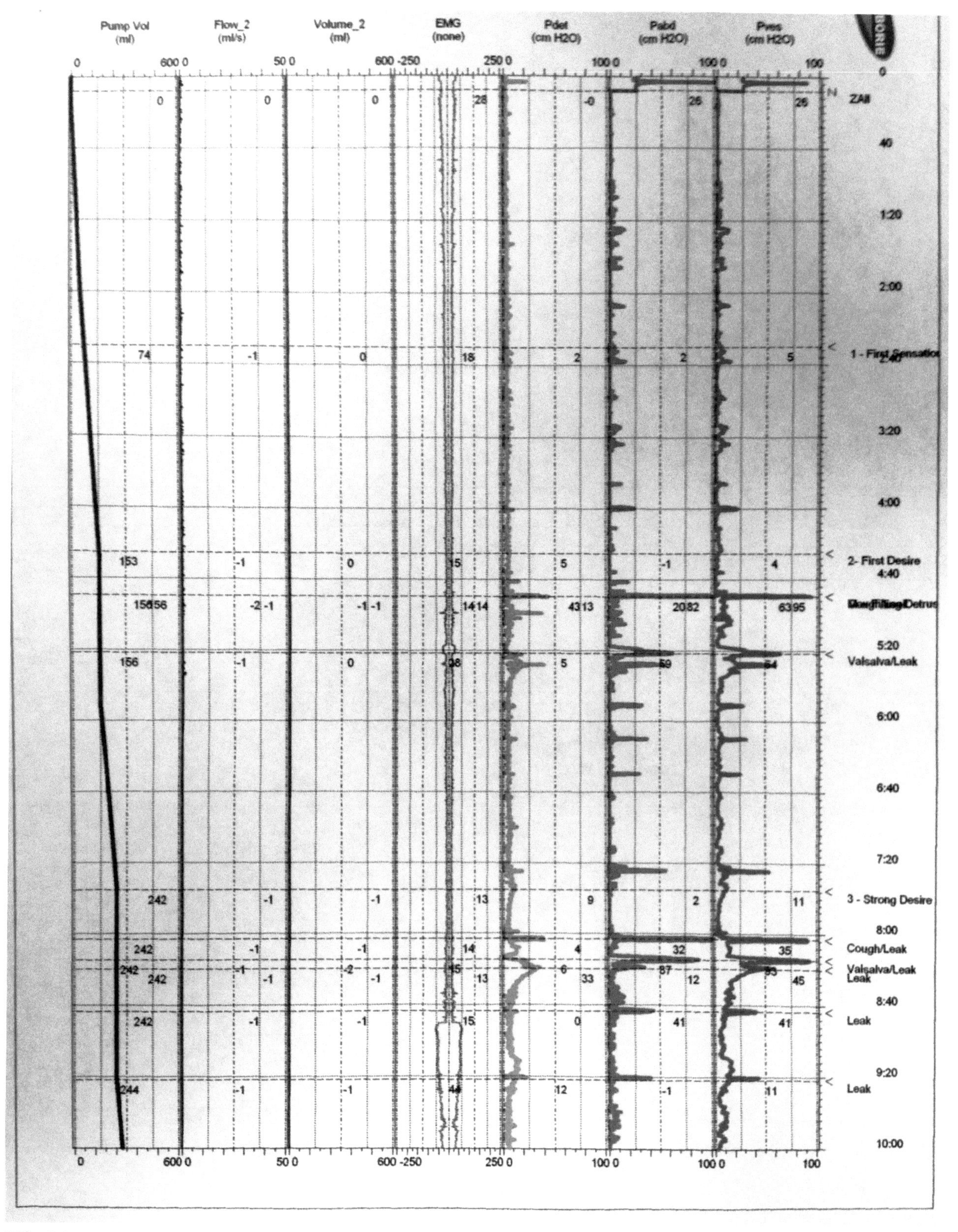

Pump Vol (ml)
Flow_2 (ml/s)
Volume_2 (ml)
EMG (none)
Pdet (cm H2O)
Pabd (cm H2O)
Pves (cm H2O)
ZAll
1 - First Sensation
2- First Desire
Valsalva/Leak
3 - Strong Desire
Cough/Leak
Valsalva/Leak
Leak
Leak
Leak
0
40
1:20
2:00
3:20
4:00
4:40
5:20
6:00
6:40
7:20
8:00
8:40
9:20
10:00

FIG. 9-1.

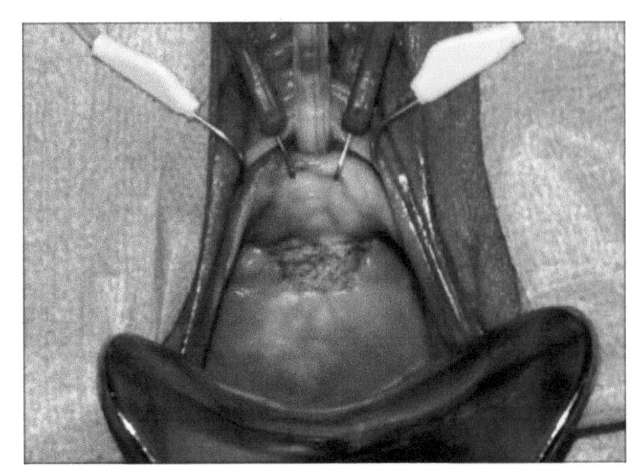

FIG. 22-1.

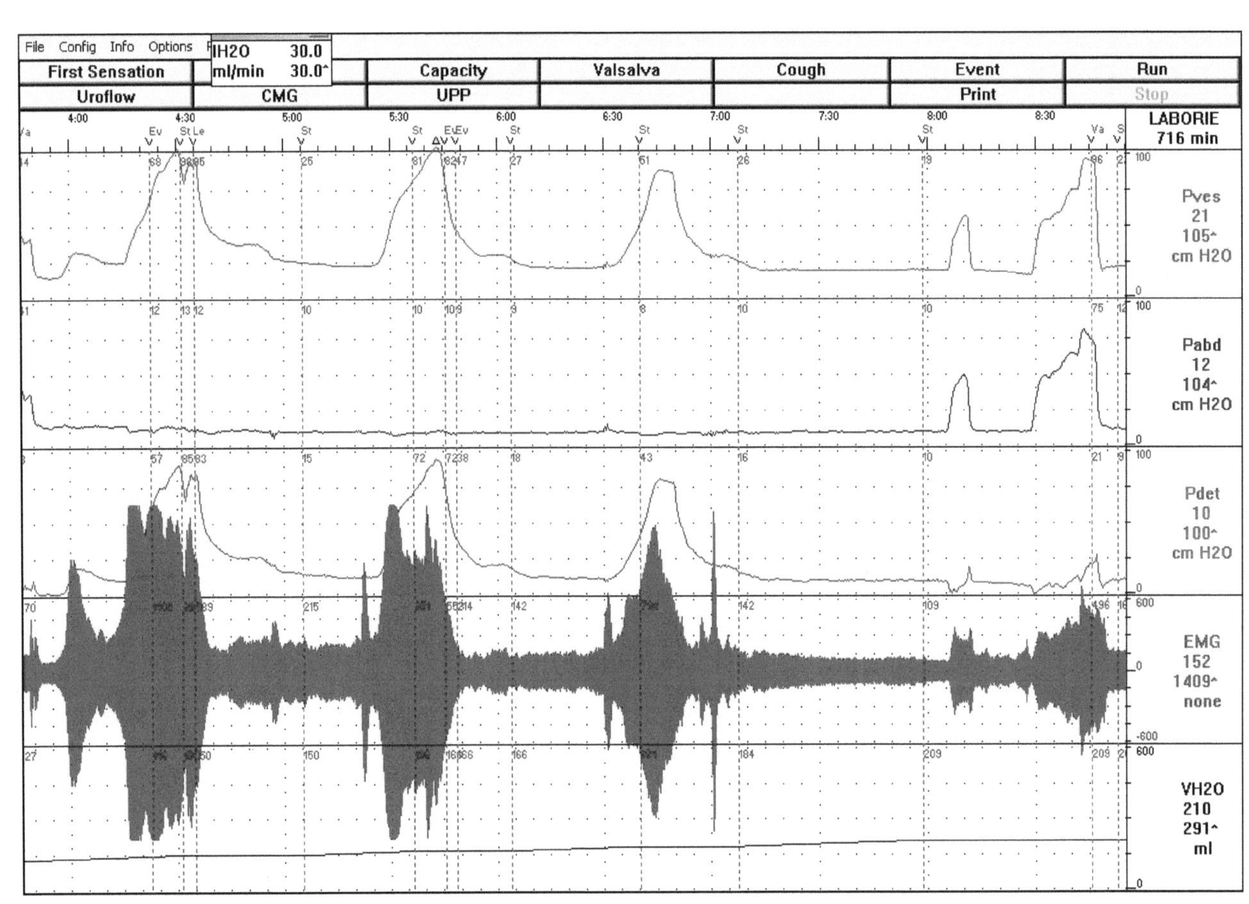

FIG. 43-1.

Acknowledgments

FIG. 9-1. Courtesy of William Stuart Reynolds, MD, Department of Urologic Surgery, Vanderbilt University Medical Center, Nashville, TN.

Fig. 22-1 was originally published in Nazemi TM, Kobashi KC. Complications of grafts used in female pelvic floor reconstruction: mesh erosion and extrusion. Indian J Urol 2007;23:153–60.

Fig. 43-1 is provided courtesy of David Ginsberg, MD, Department of Urology, University of Southern California Institute of Urology, Los Angeles, CA.